WHITE DOVE BOOKS

How to Stay Young
by Ken Strong

MY BLOG   **FREE BOOKS**   **OUR AUDIOS**   **OUR MOVIE**

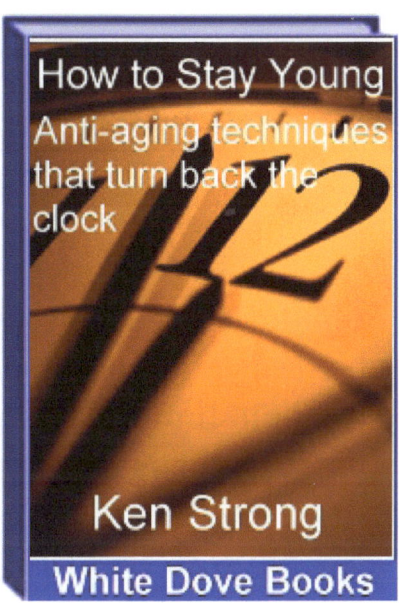

Dedicated to Uncle Gerry
Who Stayed Young & Lived Life to the Full

- You are Granted **FULL** Resale Rights to this Book
- It **MAY** be Sold or Given Away as a Bonus
- You may **NOT** alter the contents in any way
- Recommended Retail Price is: $19.97

Disclaimer

Reasonable care has been taken to ensure that the information presented in this book is accurate. However, the reader should understand that the information provided does not constitute legal, medical or professional advice of <u>any</u> kind.

No Liability: this product is supplied "as is" and without warranties. <u>All</u> warranties, express or implied, are hereby disclaimed.

Use of this product constitutes acceptance of the "No Liability" policy. If you do not agree with this policy, you are not permitted to use or distribute this product.

White Dove Books, its employees, associates, distributors, agents and affiliates shall not be liable for any losses or damages whatsoever (including, without limitation, consequential loss or damage) directly or indirectly arising from the use of this product.

Contents

The Fountain of Youth

For centuries, ever since the legendary Ponce de Leon went searching for the elusive Fountain of Youth, people have been looking for ways to slow down the aging process.

Medical science has made great strides in keeping people alive longer by preventing and curing disease, and helping people to live healthier lives. Average life expectancy keeps increasing, and most of us can look forward to the chance to live much longer lives than our ancestors.

Many researchers think that the key to our own personal Fountains of Youth resides in our hormones and endocrine system. These are the various organs and glands that make hormones in our bodies.

Yet we are all aging constantly. The unpleasant fact is that every single one of us begins aging the moment we are out of the womb - at least it beats the alternative! If you're living, you're aging; you can't avoid it. But there are a number of things that you can do to keep yourself healthy and active, and to eliminate or at least slow down many of the factors that contribute to aging.

Yes, it is possible to turn back the clock. Your body was actually designed with the inbuilt ability to fix itself, as long as you take care of it properly. Your body is made up of something like 100 *trillion* (100,000,000,000,000) living cells, which keep themselves strong and healthy with the proper food.

Each and every one of those trillions of cells dies off and is replaced with a new cell at regular intervals. Your entire body is literally completely replaced every few years – you really aren't the same person you used to be!

What happens with your cells is the key to anti-aging. When a cell dies, one of three possible things must happen:

First, if the cell has not been receiving proper nutrition, its replacement will be a weaker version of the cell. In this scenario, your body is degenerating.

The second possibility is that the replacement cell may have the same strength as its predecessor. In this case, your body essentially remains in the same place.

The third possibility is that the new cell is stronger than the previous one. Now you're actually regenerating the body, and reversing the aging process. This can only happen if you give your cells plenty of the right kind of food energy to work with.

Somewhere in our thirties, many of us start noticing those first signs that we aren't kids anymore – a few gray hairs appearing, lines in the face, skin starts sagging.

As more time goes by, other signs slowly and gradually appear – it's a little harder getting up in the morning, our vision and hearing aren't what they used to be, our sex life isn't as lively as we remember. And we look around us and see the same things apparently happening to our friends and family. Most of us pretty much automatically accept what we see as an inevitable process of nature.

Unfortunately, this is a mistake, because as the old cliché goes, you're only as old as you feel. And if you *feel* and *think* that you're getting older – well, then you are!

Your mindset does influence what goes on in your body. Meanwhile, you see your body getting older, and so you feel older, which reinforces the aging processes in your body. It becomes a vicious circle.

Fortunately, you can turn this around by using the tips and principles explained in this book. As you notice your body looking and feeling younger, your mindset will improve, which motivates you to continue your anti-aging practices, which sets up a positive feedback loop, instead of a negative one. And so the process accelerates.

People are living longer than ever these days, due to advanced medical breakthroughs, increased awareness of the importance of a healthy lifestyle, and other related factors.

The human body can take an awful lot of abuse and neglect. We don't always think about our bad habits, since it may take years or decades for the effects to become apparent. But neglect yourself long enough, and you may one day find yourself suffering through the late period of your life with a wide range of maladies and complaints, from difficulty seeing and hearing to cancer, heart disease, brittle bones, and many other problems.

Yet it only takes a little knowledge and a bit of work to prevent most, if not all, of these common old-age problems from manifesting. There's no magic pill or instant cure, and it will take some effort on your part. But the results will be well worth it -- how much would it be worth to you to enjoy your final years as a healthy, active adult, able to continue doing many of the things you most love?

How & Why We Age

Most people just shrug and accept aging as something that can't be avoided – like death and taxes. Perhaps we haven't figured out how to cheat death yet, but recent scientific discoveries have shown that common conceptions of aging are largely mistaken. For most species on the planet (as well as humans until only very recently), it was unlikely for anyone to survive long enough to die of simple "old age." Events such as starvation, accident, being eaten by a predator, disease, and other causes were the usual reason for death.

There are number of theories about exactly why and how we age. You may have heard of free radicals – a free radical is a special type of molecule with an extra electron that steals electrons from other molecules as it passes through your bloodstream, causing damage to your body's cells. The exact role of free radicals is still uncertain, and much research is still being done, but studies have established that the presence of free radicals plays a part in diseases such as Alzheimer's disease, arthritis, hypertension, and other health problems.

Studies have also shown a definite relationship between a strong and healthy response to stress and aging. Free radicals can cause progressive damage to the body's tissue and functioning, and thereby increase the rate of aging. A good stress fights off the free radicals, which in turn slows down the aging process and increases your lifespan.

There are a number of substances that function as anti-oxidants that work to bind the unstable free radicals and render them harmless. Many of these substances will be discussed further on in this book, but they include Vitamin C, Vitamin E, beta-carotene, grape seed extract, Melatonin, and other substances.

It's only in modern times, when increasing numbers of people live long enough to die from so-called "natural causes," that the role of phenomena such as free radicals has become important enough to study.

Another theory of aging focuses on how our DNA works. DNA is the blueprint of our individual body and life, and is inherited from our parents. The theory here is that our individual code ages us at a predetermined rate, possibly to keep humans from overpopulating by making sure we don't stick around too long taking up room. But this code can also be altered or "fooled" into aging much more slowly, through improving our diet and lifestyle and avoiding pollution and other environmental toxins as much as possible.

Another theory posits that the nucleic acids, or telomeres, in our cells shorten slightly every time one of our cells replicates itself. Each time the cell is duplicated, it's a less than perfect copy of the previous version, and this eventually leads to the body's aging, breakdown, and death. In other words, like your car, you can only repair the machine so many times – eventually it just simply wears out.

Scientists have recently found a direct link that indicates that excessive fat in your body speeds up the aging process. Studies found that the more that someone weighs, the older their cells are. The exact mechanism by which this process happens is still uncertain, but possibly the fat cells help weaken and destroy important genetic structures.

It was found that being overweight effectively makes a person **nine years older**, on average!

Many of the most common health problems we encounter in Western societies, such as cancer, diabetes, heart disease, and other greater and lesser maladies, may occur due to fat cells hurrying up the process of aging.

A lot of it boils down to **proper nutrition and exercise.** We know that the proper nutrition and exercise can and will make a difference on how healthy our bodies age. Just as smoking, sugar, and alcohol may not show effects for years and years but very few get away without repercussions. Cardiovascular disease, cancer, and osteoporosis are three debilitating diseases that diet and exercise can have an intense effect on. Let me share with you what we know about keeping our bodies healthy.

Exercise Need Not be Hard Work

Studies have shown that living a sedentary lifestyle actually presents a higher risk for heart disease than high cholesterol or even smoking! No matter what your age, whether you're closing in on 40, racing past 50 or 60, or older, you will improve your health and mood by exercising regularly.

Even nursing home residents in their 80s and 90s became stronger and more independent through exercise. You'll feel better and have much more energy than you did before.

Some of us are better than others at sticking to our exercise plans, but the benefits of regular physical activity are almost too numerous to list here. Regular exercise will keep excess weight off, put calcium in your bones and keep them healthy, keep your cholesterol down, make your metabolism more efficient, and help clean your body of toxins through sweating and regular bowel movements.

Even better, regular exercise strengthens your heart, lowers your cholesterol, lowers your stress, and helps you to sleep better. When you're in good physical shape, your risk of diabetes, heart disease, and even some kinds of cancer lower dramatically. It also has been shown to help reduce depression.

Sound good? And you don't have to become a marathon runner or torture yourself through an Arnold Schwarzenegger-style bodybuilding program in order to enjoy the benefits – just 30 minutes of moderate physical activity several times a week will do the trick. Just do <u>something</u> – anything to get started, even taking short walks every day.

If you've never exercised regularly, or have been sedentary for quite a while, you should have a routine medical checkup before starting any new program (just to be on the safe side!).

Once you've gotten your doctor's okay – take it slow to begin with! Slow and steady wins the race, as the old saying goes. It's much more effective to start a reasonable program that you'll actually stay with for the long run, rather than racing out of the gate like gangbusters and burning yourself out after a week. Thirty minutes a day is all you need, and it doesn't even have to be all at one time. Taking the stairs instead of using the elevator, mowing the lawn, even chores around the house, can easily add up to 30 minutes over the course of a day.

Before starting your activity, if it's going to be anything more strenuous than walking, it's a good idea to spend between 5 and 15 minutes stretching. This gives you more flexibility and ease of movement, and decreases your risk of straining your muscles or otherwise injuring yourself. A similar period of stretching after your exercise is useful for cooling yourself down and relaxing.

It's best to vary your exercise routine. Not only is this more beneficial to your health, you'll be much less likely to injure yourself or get bored. You should be working hard enough that it's difficult to carry on a normal conversation at the same time, but you shouldn't be working so hard that you're gasping for every breath.

Also try to find something that you enjoy doing. Obviously, that will make you that much more likely to continue doing it.

Try to mix these three types of exercise: **aerobic, strength,** and **flexibility.** Aerobic exercise helps to strengthen your heart, increases your lung capacity, and improves your blood circulation.

Strength conditioning helps make you stronger and increases your metabolism and bone density. Flexibility exercises, besides helping you to move more easily (obviously!), keep your joints in good shape and make it less likely that they will be stiff and painful as you get older.

One way to do this is to join your local health club. Then you'll have access to a wide range of stationary bicycles, stair-steppers, and other aerobic machines. Plus, there are usually qualified trainers on staff who can help you design a personal program that's safe and appropriate for you. But you can also do a very effective exercise program at home, either by yourself or with a friend or spouse. Then the only financial investment you'll have is for a pair of decent athletic shoes.

The better condition you are in, the more efficient your body will be at burning fat. So, while you still want to keep healthy dietary habits, if you want to lose weight it will be far more effective if you exercise regularly and eat what you like, rather than starving yourself.

How to Stop Aging

There are three types of exercise that can actually slow down, or even stop the aging process:

Aerobic

The best way to strengthen your heart muscle is through cardiovascular, or aerobic, exercise. This is activity that will get your heart rate pumped up to between 60 and 90 percent of your recommended maximum heart rate. (To figure your maximum rate, just take 220 and subtract your current age.)

While your body does burn calories constantly through normal functions such as breathing and blood circulation, if you do anything more exciting, your body needs to find some extra energy. It does this by burning <u>glycogen</u>, which is the carbohydrates and fat stored in your body. The most efficient way of burning fat is medium-intensity activities that can be done for a longer period, such as swimming or power walking.

Almost any physical activity you can do will help. Take the stairs instead of the elevator, park a little further away from your destination than usual, walk or ride your bike instead of driving. There are ways you can insert regular exercise into your regular life in an organic way – for instance, if you normally watch a lot of TV, get a stationary bicycle or a treadmill and put it in front of the TV, and use it while you're watching. Thirty minutes a day is all you really need, and three 10-minute bursts of activity will work as well as a single 30-minute workout. The key is to take action and just <u>do something</u> – it almost doesn't matter what that something is.

If you want something a bit more challenging, you can attend one of the wide varieties of aerobic dance classes at your local health club or community center. The important thing is to find the activities that you enjoy doing, and that fit your current lifestyle and fitness level.

If you have illnesses that restrict your activities, talk to your doctor – there's most likely something that you can do. For instance, if you have arthritis, swimming is a very beneficial activity that won't strain or injure your joints.

Strength

Lifting weights is a great way to build strength, become more flexible, and increase your bone density, which is especially of concern to women as they age. Increasing your muscular strength in this way will make such everyday things like climbing stairs or rising from a chair easier when you get older.

By strengthening your muscles in this way, you have more energy and better posture; you're less likely to suffer muscle-related tears or other injuries; and you will look and feel more attractive.

In addition, building muscle mass increases your metabolism rate, which means you burn fat more efficiently, without going on any unhealthy crash diets. (You may not weigh less after lifting weights for a while, but an increasing amount of your body fat will be transformed into muscle!) Weight training also lowers your cholesterol, reduces stress, and helps prevent a wide variety of diseases.

There are a variety of brands and types of equipment that are commonly used in weight training, from individual dumbbells or barbells to freestanding machines. There are pros and cons of each type of training, although a lot of it will come down to personal preference and what works best for you.

In any strength-training program, the number one concern is always your safety. If you haven't done any weight training before, take it easy at the beginning. Machines with adjustable resistance are the best place to start out. This gives you the chance to work on specific, isolated muscle groups of your choice, and also lets you keep track of your progress, by slowly increasing the weight and resistance that you're lifting.

On the other hand, free weights tend to develop your strength more quickly. They develop more muscles at once, as opposed to resistance machines that isolate single muscle groups.

Free weights are more versatile, since you're not restricted to the machine's specific motions, although as a result, more coordination is needed to use free weights safely and effectively. Free weights are also much cheaper than machines (if you're purchasing them for personal use rather than joining a health club), and take up much less space when you're not using them.

The ideal strength-training program would involve a combination of free weights and resistance machines. If you belong to a health club, there most likely are trainers on staff who can help you develop a personalized strength-training program that's best suited for you.

Flexibility

Of the three main types of exercise, flexibility is most likely to get overlooked by most people. The benefits from aerobic and strength training are fairly obvious (lose weight, build muscles and strength, get fit generally), but flexibility has its own important part to play, even if its benefits are less obvious.

As you age, however, you will learn more and more to appreciate the benefits you get by regular stretching and other flexibility exercises. Keeping flexible keeps you more limber and makes many ordinary day-to-day activities much easier and more enjoyable. Being more flexible also helps prevent many kinds of injuries.

If you belong to a health club or otherwise can get access to a qualified personal trainer or physical therapist, you can work out a stretching program tailored to your individual needs, much more beneficial than doing a few generic stretches.

Stretching helps get rid of the tension in your body. Many of us habitually hold tension in various parts of our bodies, often without even being consciously aware of it. The most common tense areas are the chest, shoulder, hamstrings, and hips. When doing any kind of stretching, pay attention to what your body is telling you. Take it slow and easy, especially if you are older, pregnant, or if you are suffering from any kind of injury or disability.

Yoga is an increasingly common practice for people attracted to its many physical, mental, and psychological benefits. There are many different types of yoga, but generally it refers to a system of stretching exercises that improve the functioning of your body's circulatory, respiratory, and digestive systems, as well as making the body stronger and more flexible. Many people also say that regular yoga practice brings them increased clarity and peace of mind and more emotional stability.

The idea behind yoga is that the health of your spine determines your real age – regular yoga practice keeps your spine flexible, firms up your skin, keeps your chin single (and not double or triple), and helps tone your body and improve your posture. You're only as old as you feel, and if your body looks and feels younger than your years, then you *are* younger than your years.

Doing yoga postures stretches your body in many ways and increases the blood flow to areas of your body that don't always get enough. Your brain and other internal organs will like the increased oxygen that comes from the improved blood circulation. Besides the immediate benefits to your well-being, a regular yoga practice will keep you active and alert in your older years.

Besides the actual physical stretches and postures, a typical yoga class may also include instruction on better breathing, and using various meditation and visualization techniques that help your mind and body to function together at a higher level.

Another popular type of exercise widely taught in classes is the Pilates system, named after its originator, Joseph Pilates. The system dates from the time of World War I, when Pilates wanted to improve the health and morale of his fellow soldiers. Later on, he added the use of resistance springs, and then developed the machines and other equipment now commonly used in Pilates classes. For years the system was mainly used by professional dancers, until the 1980s, when Pilates became widely popular through classes at health clubs and community centers.

The key goal of the Pilates program is to help you improve your mental focus, learn muscle control, and make movements more efficiently and effectively. Some of the ways this is achieved include learning to align your spine properly, strengthening your back and abdomen muscles to promote the healthiest posture, and using your breath to calm and focus your mind and reduce mental chatter.

Eating to Stay Young

Looking and feeling younger is a lot more under your control than you may think. A lot of the signs of aging that we assume are natural and unavoidable, such as wrinkles, decreasing mobility, less acute sight and hearing, disease, and assorted chronic aches and pains, come in large part from not taking proper care of ourselves. The choices you make when feeding yourself are just as important as exercise and other elements of your anti-aging strategy.

Studies have shown that putting lots of fresh fruits and vegetables into your diet gives you more energy, helps manage your weight, and lowers your risk for many diseases. The reasons for this include the fact that most fruits and vegetables have no fat or cholesterol, and they are low in calories, which means you can fill yourself up without gaining weight.

Produce also contains lots of fiber, which helps prevent cancer, diabetes, high blood pressure, and heart disease. They are also filled with important vitamins and minerals, including Vitamin C, folic acid, iron, calcium, and beta-carotene.

Fruits and vegetables are also chock full of antioxidants (discussed in Chapter 1), which get rid of those destructive free radicals that attack and damage our cells. Eating a diet that contains plenty of antioxidants is a good way to combat aging, in addition to preventing many types of disease. Antioxidants also build up the immune system, help prevent heart disease, and reduce the risk of prostate cancer in men.

Another aspect of a healthy anti-aging diet is to simply eat less. Numerous studies have shown that people who don't eat at every meal until they're stuffed live significantly longer and have much lower rates of all those lovely age-related diseases you've heard me mention so many times already, such as heart disease, cancer, diabetes, and many others. (They bear repeating, because the stakes are so high here!)

But when I say eat less, that doesn't mean starving yourself or neglecting to eat the right kinds of food. Decrease your portions of sugar, fat, fast food, and other empty calories, but consume plenty of fresh fruits and vegetables, legumes, and whole grains.

Eat less red meat, and more fish. Fish are rich in a good kind of fat, the omega-3 fatty acids, which are good for your heart and your immune system. Omega-3 also helps prevent the growth of cancer cells.

Fruits, vegetables, and many plant extracts also have chemicals called phytonutrients, which help keep your skin looking nice and healthy. The role of phytonutrients in plants includes giving them their color, repelling insect enemies, and attracting bees for pollination. (Antioxidants are a type of phytonutrient.)

Another aspect of good health that will keep you young longer is a healthy digestive system and colon, including regular bowel movements. While not the most glamorous of topics, it's still vitally important. When John Wayne was autopsied after his death from lung and stomach cancer, over 40 pounds of hard fecal matter was found stuck to the sides of his intestines! Keeping yourself regular prevents this from happening to your insides.

The best ways to promote good digestion and elimination are to get regular exercise, drink plenty of water every day, and eat a good diet with plenty of fiber. Other obstacles to a healthy colon include high levels of stress, a sudden change in your daily routine, pregnancy, and taking certain medications.

The Nutrition You Need

Vitamins are organic nutrients, usually separated into two categories: water-soluble, which includes the B vitamin group and Vitamin C, and fat-soluble, which includes Vitamins A, D, E, & K.

When you take fat-soluble vitamins, they get stored in your body's fat tissues until the body needs them. They may wait in your tissues for anywhere from a few days to six months. The water-soluble group of vitamins stays in your bloodstream, and any unused part is quickly eliminated in your urine, so the water-soluble vitamins need to be replenished much more often.

When we get older, generally our bodies find it more difficult to process the nutrients we put into it. We can make up for this inefficiency with the intelligent use of various vitamins, minerals, and other anti-aging supplements.

Vitamin A: Vitamin A keeps your skin and mucous membranes strong and resistant to viruses and bacteria. It also helps keep your immune system strong.

Vitamin B: Our bodies become less efficient at absorbing the B vitamins as we age, so taking supplements is a good idea. Three specific B vitamins are especially important to your health: B6, B12, and folic acid. Deficiencies in these vitamins raise your risk for heart disease and loss of memory. Recommended daily doses are 5mg of Vitamin B6, 10mcg of Vitamin B12, and 400mcg of folic acid. Pregnant women should double their dose of folic acid.

Vitamin D: Getting enough Vitamin D is a good way to prevent osteoporosis. Being out in the sunlight is one way to get Vitamin D in a natural and enjoyable way, but as we grow older, our bodies absorb it less efficiently and we need supplemental amounts. A daily dose between 400 IU and 600 IU should be sufficient.

Vitamin E: Vitamin E is an excellent antioxidant, and helps lower your blood pressure.

<u>Vitamin K:</u> Vitamin K is thought to be an even stronger antioxidant than Vitamin E. A good place to find naturally occurring Vitamin K is in green leafy vegetables, or it can be taken as a supplement. Vitamin K is unique among the fat-soluble group of vitamins in that it is not stored in the body.

<u>Amino Acids:</u> There are only 22 different amino acids, divided into two groups called **essential amino acids** and **nonessential amino acids**. They combine into long protein chains that produce the various enzymes and hormones necessary to the healthy functioning of all your essential body organs, including your heart, brain, liver, and kidneys.

The essential amino acids do not occur naturally in the body, and must be obtained through eating protein-rich foods. The nonessential amino acids are made within the body by combining two or more essential amino acids.

Since so many of us eat diets that include a lot of processed foods, which often do not contain the right kinds of protein that provide amino acids, a lot of people can benefit from taking amino acid supplements.

Coenzyme Q10 (CoQ10): This enzyme helps turn fats and sugars into energy. As you get older, you have much less CoQ10 in your body. It's essential to have plenty of it for healthy cellular growth.

Green Tea: Green tea has many benefits – it helps keep the DNA of cells intact, it helps prevent cancer cells from developing, and it's an excellent antioxidant (one cup of green tea has more antioxidant power than a serving of spinach, carrots, or broccoli).

Fish Oil: As noted earlier in our chapter on Nutrition, fish are a good source of a good kind of fat called omega-3 fatty acids. Besides eating fish, you can get this important fish oil in capsule form. Fish oil has been shown to reduce the risk of heart disease by promoting healthy blood flow in your body. Flaxseed oil and primrose oil also give you similar benefits.

Garlic: Garlic builds your immunity, helps prevent infections, lowers your cholesterol and blood pressure, and reduces your risk of contracting colon or stomach cancer. It can either be eaten directly as a food seasoning, or taken in capsule form.

Spirulina: Spirulina is a type of blue-green algae that grows in the water in warm parts of the world, including Africa, Hawaii, and Central America. Spirulina is an excellent source of protein, and contains all of the essential amino acids. It also is a strong antioxidant and helps prevent cancer. And if that's not enough, spirulina is also good for your immune system and lowers your cholesterol.

The Silent Killer

Stress by itself is not necessarily bad – depending on how much stress and how we react to it. Too much stress contributes to a lot of our physical ailments, including cancer, heart disease, and many other diseases. Our psychological well-being is also threatened by stress, which can cause anxiety and depression, among other mental problems.

Stress comes from many sources – financial problems, relationship problems, stress at work, fighting traffic, noise, even getting ready for a vacation. People react to stress in different ways, and some handle it better than others. Too much stress can cause you to be tired all the time, depressed, and withdrawn. You might develop skin problems or other annoying physical symptoms, get headaches and digestive problems, and lose your appetite and your sex drive.

Another common source of stress is major life events, such as divorce, the death of a spouse or other loved one, losing your job, or even just a major change of your daily routine. Too many of these major events in too short of a time may give you significant physical or psychological symptoms.

The body reacts to stress by releasing hormones that have the effect of lowering your white blood cell count, which in turn weakens your immune system. This process is more commonly known as the "fight or flight" response. Even though the overwhelming majority of us seldom if ever find ourselves in a truly life-threatening situation, our bodies become accustomed to being in a constant state of low-grade emergency response. This takes its toll over time.

There are a number of proven methods for relieving excess stress, all of which also help with the anti-aging process. One is exercise, which we've already talked about earlier. Even a simple walk will help relax you and clear your mind.

Here are some other relaxation methods:

Deep breathing: It may sound ridiculous to say that you need to learn how to breathe, but many of us have unconsciously learned poor and inefficient breathing habits, learned from years of being constantly stressed out. When you are feeling especially anxious, just find a comfortable place to sit, and take slow, deep breaths. Count slowly from 1 to 4 while you inhale, and then exhale just as slowly, again counting to four. Do this for a few minutes, and the extra oxygen in your body will make you feel relaxed and refreshed.

Visualization: To rephrase an old cliché, you are what you think. Try and catch yourself next time you start thinking anxious, angry, or otherwise negative thoughts. Your emotions follow your thoughts, and you will begin to *feel* anxious, angry, and negative. To counteract this, find a comfortable, quiet place to sit, close your eyes, and see in your mind's eye a place (either real or imagined) that makes you feel relaxed, safe, and happy. It doesn't really matter what you imagine, as long as it makes you feel good. As your mind calms down, your body will, too.

In addition, you can put on a CD, tape, or MP3 of relaxing music while you're visualizing.

Meditation: Meditation is a huge subject that we'll cover fairly briefly here – you can find plenty of additional information and techniques online or at your local library. Various forms of meditation have been used around the world for thousands of years. Frequently, it has been part of religious and spiritual practices, but you can also use it for simple relaxation and stress reduction.

Meditation really isn't all that complicated. The main idea is that you consciously relax your entire body while concentrating all of your mental focus, like a laser beam, on one thing. This focus can be on an object (such as a burning candle, for instance), or a sound, or even your own breath. The main goal is to concentrate on the chosen thing for a sustained period of time. This keeps your mind occupied and helps quiet down the incessant monkey-like chatter that normally occupies our minds from the moment we awake in the morning until we fall asleep at night. You become calmer and your body gets a chance to recuperate from the everyday stresses.

Some ways to get started meditating:

- **Find a meditation technique or style that fits your personality and doesn't conflict with your beliefs.** You can incorporate a meditation session into a yoga or tai chi routine, or use it as part of your morning and evening prayers.

- **Make meditation a set part of your day and your life.** Take it slow and easy at the beginning. You're doing well if you can do it for five minutes once or twice a day. As you get comfortable with the procedure, work your way gradually up to 20 minutes at a time. You can set a clock nearby within your peripheral vision, or set an alarm that's not too loud and jarring.

- **Be persistent, the results may not happen instantly.** Take it easy on yourself, too. It doesn't make too much sense to get stressed out at yourself because you're not relaxing quickly enough! While you're trying to concentrate on your chosen object, your mind will inevitably wander constantly. That's fine; just gently return your focus to the object.

Meditation is one of the simplest and cheapest therapeutic stress-reduction techniques around. You can do it anytime. It just requires a little bit of time and practice.

Now It's Up to You

The nice thing about all the anti-aging techniques given in this book is that you can use any of them individually, and it will make a difference in your life. But if you use more than one of them, or all of them, the effect is much greater than the sum of the individual parts. There is a synergistic effect, with each technique in your strategy mutually and simultaneously strengthening the others.

Eating right gives you more energy, which makes you feel more like exercising, which gives you even more energy, which reduces your stress and relaxes you, which makes meditation that much more effective…you get the idea. You should have plenty of ideas now about how you can slow down, halt, and even reverse the aging process in your body and mind.

Good luck, good health, and have a long and happy life!

About White Dove Books

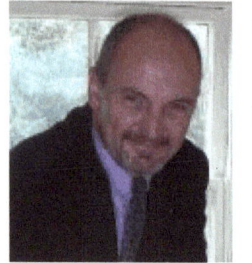 Will Edwards is the founder of <u>White Dove Books</u> - the internet's leading website for Self Improvement and Personal Development. A graduate of the University of Birmingham (UK) he develops and teaches Personal Development workshops and he is a published author.

Within its first three years, White Dove Books was recognised as one of the internet's leading sites for self help and personal development; breaking into the top 100,000 sites on the internet at the end of 2005.

The INSPIRATION newsletter was started in 2005 as a way of providing helpful information including tips, articles and free inspirational ebooks to our visitors.

Today White Dove Books works in partnership with many authors and on-line publishers of inspirational material to provide a quality on-line service that serves thousands of people in many countries across the world.

Our mission is to help people to develop their own unique talents, abilities and passion in order that they may lead more meaningful, joyful and fulfilled lives

The Personal Success Series

The Deepest Desire of Your Heart

by Will Edwards

Find & Fulfil Your Unique Purpose in Life

Using the exact methods taught in our program, very many people are already producing amazing results in their lives; and so can you.

Our outstanding program represents the culmination of many years of research into the application of the principles of success; and everything you need to accomplish the most amazing transformation of your life is included.

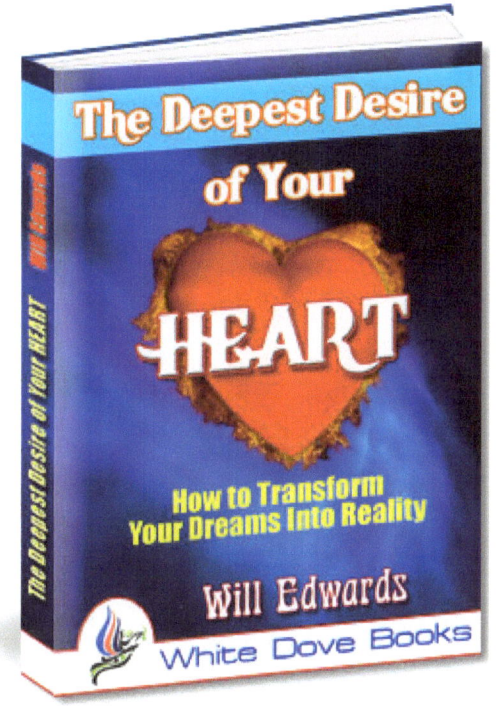

☑ **Discover Your Unique Calling**

☑ **Stay On-Track to Achieve Your Mission**

☑ **Overcoming Obstacles**

☑ **Getting from Theory to Making it Happen**

☑ **Professional Tips & Exercises**

☑ **Identify Your Most Important Activities**

☑ **Complete System to Optimize Time**

☑ **How to Ensure You Achieve Your Goals**

Click Here for More Details …

The Personal Success Series

The 7 Keys to Success
by Will Edwards

Your FREE Gift from White Dove Books!

The 7 Keys to Success began as a Movie at the White Dove Books site. We then made it into an eCourse for our subscribers. Now finally, it is available as a <u>FREE</u> eBook.

This book contains an important message. I hope you will get your copy and work with us to change the world.

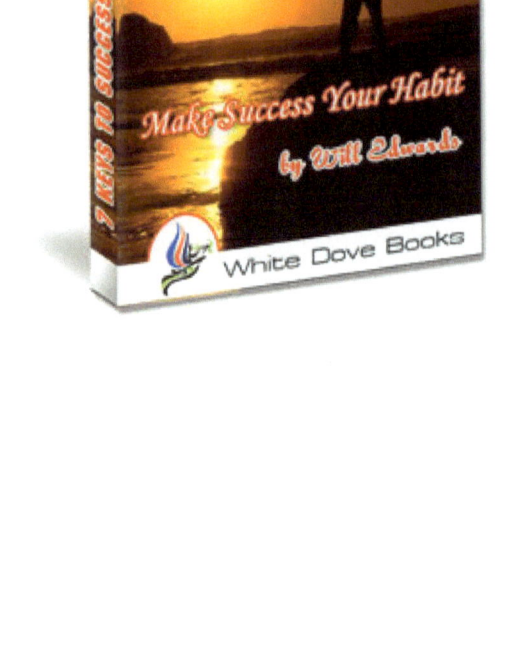

☑ **Commitment**

☑ **An Open Mind**

☑ **Persistence**

☑ **Flexibility**

☑ **Faith**

☑ **Thankfulness**

☑ **Passion**

☑ **INCLUDED** – You may give away this book as a free gift to your friends. You may use it as a free bonus. It may NOT be sold. You can help us to make a real difference by getting this important message to the people of the world.

<u>Click Here</u> for More Details …

The Guru's Apprentice Series

How the Jerk Got Rich
by Will Edwards

How to use <u>Subliminal</u> Techniques to Write a Sales Page that Sells!

The first book in the *Guru's Apprentice* series deals with the techniques used by the infamous Rich Jerk. It shows exactly what you need to do to make the breakthrough and reach financial independence.

This cutting-edge report deals with the results of our earliest testing of the Rich Jerk's principles. You will find out exactly how the Rich Jerk used advanced subliminal techniques to market his products and how you can do the same.

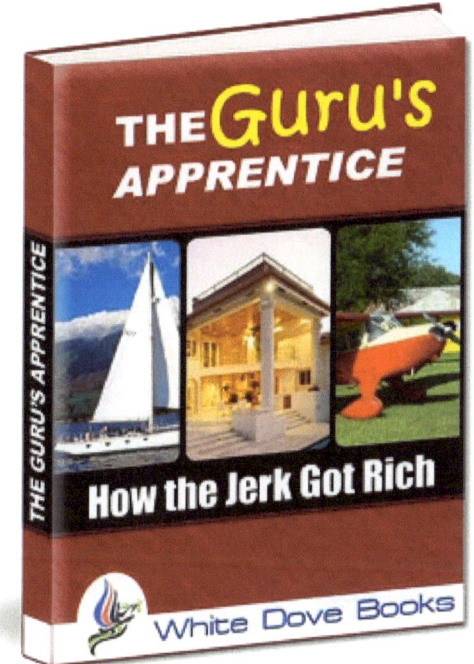

☑ **INCLUDED** - *How the Jerk Got Rich* book revealing the subliminal techniques the Rich Jerk has used to generate **massive** on-line profit - secret techniques you can legally copy!

☑ **INCLUDED** - A Professionally written Sales Page complete with Professional Graphics - the cost of these graphics alone is far greater than the very small price of this offer.

☑ **INCLUDED** - Master Resale Rights to the book *How the Jerk Got Rich.* You may resell this book and keep 100% of the profits. You may also sell the Resale Rights for pure profit.

Click Here for More Details …

The Guru's Apprentice Series

Protect Your Product
by Will Edwards

How to Combat Copyright Theft of <u>YOUR</u> Digital Products

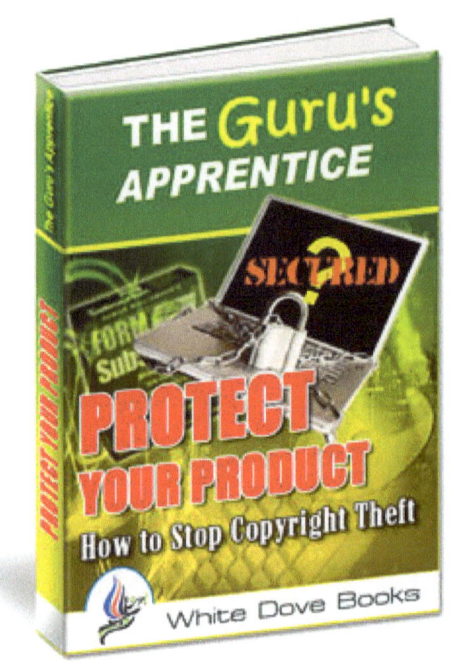

Do you know what is the biggest problem Internet Marketers are facing today? It is Copyright Infringement. That's when someone else steals your product and robs you of the profit that is rightfully yours!

It is a growing problem for writers and publishers of digital products! In this book you will find a simple, workable solution to the problem.

✔ **INCLUDED** - *How to Fight Copyright Theft* revealing the simple 6-Step system anyone can use to protect original work without paying for registration services.

✔ **INCLUDED** - Professionally written Sales Page complete with Professional Graphics - the cost of these graphics alone is far greater than the very small price of this offer.

✔ **INCLUDED** - Master Resale Rights to the book *How to Fight Copyright Theft*. You may resell this book and keep 100% of the profits. You may also sell the Master Resale Rights for pure profit.

<u>Click Here</u> for More Details ...